In Search
of Recovery:
A Christian Man's Guide

In Search of Recovery:

A Christian Man's Guide

Clinical Guide

Paul Becker, LPC

authorHOUSE®

AuthorHouse™
1663 Liberty Drive
Bloomington, IN 47403
www.authorhouse.com
Phone: 1-800-839-8640

Published by AuthorHouse   01/25/2012

ISBN: 978-1-4685-4794-8 (sc)
ISBN: 978-1-4685-4793-1 (e)

This book: *In Search of Recovery: A Clinical Guide,* is written for therapists/counselors for use in a clinical environment. It is an instructional guide on how to use the books;

In Search of Recovery: A Christian Man's Guide and

In Search of Recovery Workbook: A Christian Man's Guide

These books help men to remove unwanted sexual behavior from their lives.

Both Christian Man's Guide books may be purchased from Gentle Path Press or directly/ on-line from: sexaddiction.sexaddictionhelpbooks.com

Contents

Introduction

This guide is intended to facilitate the use of the book, *In Search of Recovery: A Christian Man's Guide* and the accompanying workbook in a sex addiction group program. It supports clinical therapists by providing interventions for men who wish to end addictive sexual behaviors. This intervention program can be summarized through the following statements: Vision, Program Goal and Objectives of Therapy.

Leading Vision: Assist men who are seeking God in the right places.

Program Goal: Men who participate in this program will end lustful sexual thinking, fantasies and behavior.

Program Objective: Lead men through a structured clinical process intended to help them become aware and understand the complex factors that contribute to sexual addiction. The program objective is supported by exploring:

- The nature, characteristics, and factors underlying sexual addiction will be respectfully addressed.

- The beginning of sexual addiction is most often found in age-inappropriate exposure to sexual behavior or material.

- Age-inappropriate exposure to sexual behavior or material causes feelings of sexual arousal, shame, and guilt. These confusing feelings together with a lack of fatherly emotional nourishment often form the roots of sexual addiction.

- Sexual addiction is a shame-based disease that began at a time in life when adult choices were not possible. The addict is not a bad person but is dealing with a bad problem.

- Each sexually addicted man is not alone in his struggle; a substantial proportion of the male population struggles with the elements of sexual addiction at some time during their lives.

- The challenges of overcoming compulsive addictive behavior are addressed through educational and behavioral modification processes.

- Anger, anxiety, depressed mood, and isolation contribute to lustful thinking, fantasies, and behavior.

- By empowering men to exercise choice there is hope of changing the sexual addiction dance.

- Recovery includes changing one's attachment to sexual fantasy, thinking, and behavior.

- Recovery includes changing one's life by coming out of isolation, taking steps to give up depressed mood, improving family relationships, and developing a support network.

- God's great love and Grace can help men make a sustained, high-level commitment to end lustful sexual thinking, fantasies, and behavior.

- Many resources are available to support an addiction-free life journey.

Notes:

This program is spiritually based but experience has taught that at the beginning of therapy most sexually addicted men have a tenuous relationship with Christ. For many men it takes time to change how they think about themselves and thus how they relate to God. Dealing with shame and guilt and finding the blessing of self-respect are prerequisites to understanding the great love that Christ has for all his people, including the sexually addicted man.

At least a twenty to twenty-five-weekly sessions are needed to lead sexually addicted men through the text and accompanying workbook, *In Search of Recover: A Christian Man's Guide.* This estimate is based on ninety minutes sessions.

This guide is not intended to be definitive in terms of the time needed to process each concept. The goal is not to complete the book and workbook. Working at the pace of the group is far more important. As such, it is within reason to add more sessions to your program. At times the counselor will find it prudent to attend to one or more unplanned agendas brought to the session by group members. Little or no progress is made in the text or workbook during some sessions. Also, adding supplemental material to the program is often helpful to the progress of the group.

All group members should be encouraged to attend a Twelve Step Program. Appendix A of the book, *In Search of Recover: A Christian Man's Guide*, lists Twelve Step Programs for sexually addicted men.

Completing the book and workbook will not assure universal cessation of sexually acting-out behavior. Each man progresses on his own internal timetable. For some, ending acting-out behavior comes quickly. But for many, progress is considerably slower. It is not usual for men to repeat the program. Addiction experts Patrick Carnes and John Bradshaw believe the healing process spans years. At the conclusion of the program all group members are encouraged to continue their healing journey through individual and marital counseling.

Some considerations for mental health professionals (referred to as counselor):

- This program has been developed for men. There is no clinical experience to suggest that this particular program is effective for women.

- Before a man attends his first group session, schedule one or more individual therapy sessions to determine whether the potential new member will contribute to and benefit by the group process. During these individual sessions encourage the man to disclose the full scope of his sexual history and current acting-out behavior. During the group program, while men are encouraged to disclose the nature of their acting-out behavior, they are not encouraged to provide details that may be toxic to another man in the group. In some cases, full disclosure during the group process may become a source of new behavior for a member of the group. Certain aberrant behaviors such as sex with animals or children go beyond reasonable norms of group disclosure. Certain sexual behaviors are best processed during one-on-one therapy. Keep in mind, you may be legally obligated to report sexual behavior that involves children.

- Consistent weekly, on-time attendance is an important task for group members. Establish a policy that members pay for unexcused absences.

- It is not unusual for one or more of the group members to have a public persona. Group members need to guarantee confidentiality to their fellow travelers.

- It is desirable to have a sufficient number of group members at the beginning of the program so that the group can be closed to new members. However, a man who enters the program after it has begun can still gain insights to help him change his sexual behavior. If a man enters the group halfway through the program, encourage him to stay with the program when the next series of sessions begins.

- A useful program element is to dedicate the first part of the session to "check-in." During check-in each man is invited to share his status on his healing journey. Early on in the program the dialog is between the group member and the clinical counselor. After cohesion is formed in the group, crosstalk can be helpful.

- The ideal approach is for group members to read assigned materials between sessions and discuss important concepts during the session. Unfortunately, the "ideal" doesn't always happen. It can be helpful to ask group members to sequentially read aloud chapter material during the session. After every few paragraphs or at the end of a subsection, ask members a question about the material just read. For example, "Did you identify with . . . ?" or "Share your feelings about . . ." Sometimes the discussion is short, but at other times the group strikes a golden understanding. Go with the gold!

- Despite encouragement and promises, workbook assignments are not always completed between sessions. It may it be necessary for some men to come early before each weekly session to complete workbook assignments. A less preferable option is to allot time to complete workbook exercises during a group session.

- The workbook requires men to disclose information they may find embarrassing and shameful. Some fear others or family members may read the answers they provide. You may decide to have the workbook exercises completed just prior to the session or during a session and to collect the workbooks at the end of each session and give them back at the following session. If you retain member's workbooks between sessions, confidentiality should be pledged. It is more important for each man to get in touch with the full range of his past and addictive practices than updating the counselor's knowledge, at least early on in the program. It takes time to lift the veil of shame.

- The majority of men enter therapy because their sexual behavior has been "found-out" by their spouses. It is common and understandable for a spouse to react harshly to learning that her partner has not respected the marriage vow. In these situations encourage the couple to schedule a joint therapy session. During the session empower the spouse to ask questions about sexual addiction.

- Men and women see the world differently. Sexually addicted men are driven to repeat the good feelings associated with "orgasm," whereas women see sex as part of a "relationship" commitment. A woman, rightfully, cannot understand how her partner can "do his own thing," and be committed to the marriage. The woman, indeed, has the correct concept but, on the other hand, it will take him time to alter his thinking. Ask her to give you time to work with her partner and to give him time to heal. In time, hopefully, he will see the world the same way as she does.

- Frequently, sexually addicted men have codependent marriages. Suggest to couples that the man needs an accountability partner to whom he is not married. Each partner needs time to work on his or her own issues. Freeing the spouse of the burden of accountability is often a blessing.

- Men often feel that once they have pleaded sorrow for their behavior, trust should be restored to the marriage. The couple needs to understand that ending unwanted sexual behavior is rarely an instant decision and that trust is only gained through prolonged sobriety and changed lifestyle. Encourage spouses to read *In Search of Recovery: A Christian Man's Guide, Don't Call It Love*, by Patrick Carnes, and *Getting the Love You Want, by Harville* Hendrix.

Note: For the sexually addicted man, much of the information in *In Search of Recovery: A Christian Man's Guide* and its accompanying workbook, is new to him. Certain important concepts are treated more than once. It takes more than one pass to internalize and apply important new concepts.

A syllabus for a twenty-week group therapy program follows. It is intended to be a fluid guide that can be revised and extended to suit the needs to the group.

Group Program
Session One

Goal: Introduction of the program	Material needed: Handout—2 Corinthians 12:7-10
Objective: Establish group norms and begin to expose shame.	Introduction to Group Program

Begin with a Prayer

Brief discussion of consent and disclosure form: Ask each person to sign your form.

Brief discussion of the group norms and process:

- Discuss attendance, participation, being on-time, expressing feelings, respectful confrontation, honesty, use of "I" statements ("I feel disrespected when people start whispering while I'm talking."), disclosure, dominating discussion vs. holding back, intellectualizing, confidentiality (what is said in the room stays in the room), disclosure of sensitive information about self, roles of a group leader (teacher, counselor/therapist, and supporter), and cost of the group sessions.

- The group program is a combination of education and therapy. It is not a Twelve Step program. All group members are encouraged to attend a relevant sex addiction Twelve Step program. See Appendix A in the book for a listing.

- The program structure is a combination of understanding self and the nature of sexual addiction, and how one can change one's life to reduce the influence of addiction.

- Therapeutic expectations: Ask group members to be patient and trust in the process. Unwanted sexual behavior did not begin overnight and healing will take time. For some, it may take the rest of their lives. We don't talk in terms of a cure, but in terms of a recovery journey.

- Healing takes commitment and much work. In order to cover much ground, homework should be assigned. It is essential, as a first commitment, group members should complete the assignments with considerable thought—not in the car on the way to the session.

Discuss how addictions come in various shapes and sizes. What is important is how the addiction affects an individual's life. Ask group members not to compare themselves to others. No one has an accurate measuring stick. If another man has a sexual behavior problem greater than yours—pray for him.

Introductions: Pair each man with another. Ask members to exchange information in order to report to the whole group about their partner. Ask the men to report on the following information: name, something important about the person and a personal goal the person has for group counseling. Record goals on large sheets of paper or on a white board.

Draw feelings: Ask each man to take a piece of paper and draw on one half a symbol or picture of how he feels as he comes into the group. On the other half, draw a symbol or picture how he hopes to feel after he ends his acting-out behaviors. Ask group members to share their thinking and feelings.

Discussion of humanness: We are not alone in our failings—several of the apostles had great difficulties. Ask the men to discuss their understanding of 2 Corinthians 12:7-10:

> *To keep me from becoming conceited because of these surpassingly great revelations, there was given me a thorn in my flesh, a messenger of Satan, to torment me. Three times I pleaded with the Lord to take it away from me. But he said to me, "My grace is sufficient for you, for my power is made perfect in weakness." Therefore I will boast all the more gladly about my weaknesses, so that Christ's power may rest on me. That is why, for Christ's sake, I delight in weaknesses, in insults, in hardships, in persecutions, in difficulties. For when I am weak, then I am strong.*

St. Paul, who wrote the above words, had his "thorn" in his side. We don't know what the thorn represented but we do know it troubled St. Paul — could it have been an addiction?

Between-session assignment: Ask each man to describe in writing two choices he currently faces. What are the factors affecting his choices? Include one choice related to sexual behavior. Ask group members to be prepared to discuss alternative answers at the next session.

Handouts: 2 Corinthians 12:7-10.

Homework assignment: Read Chapter One of the book, *In Search of Recovery: A Christian Man's Guide*

End with a prayer. (Suggest the Serenity Prayer) See page **53** of the book.

Group Program
Sessions Two and Three

Goal: Educate	Material needed: Book, *In Search of Recovery: A Christian Man's Guide*
Objective: Provide an understanding of sexual addiction and its characteristics.	Chapter: One

Begin with a Prayer

Report on between-session assignment: Ask each man to report on two choices he is facing and what his alternatives are. Include one choice related to sexual behavior. What are the factors affecting his choices?

From Chapter One of the book:

Page #	Action: Read and discuss.	
1-3 Book	**Primary Topic:** What Is Sexual Addiction?	The purpose of this section is to introduce the concept of sexual addiction.
	Discussion topic:	**Discussion Points:**
	What is sexual addiction?	Ask group members: To share their feelings when they hear the term "sexual addiction." If they identify with any of the material presented?

From Chapter One of the book:

Page #	**Action:** Read and discuss.	
3-4 Book	**Primary Topic:** Common Characteristics of Unwanted Sexual Behavior.	The purpose of this section is to introduce some common characteristics of unwanted sexual behavior.
	Discussion topics:	**Discussion Points:**
3 Book	Multiple practices.	No discussion is needed.
3 Book	Practices become compulsive and unmanageable.	Ask group members to share how their sexual behavior has become unmanageable.
3 Book	Life-damaging consequences.	Ask group members to share the negative consequences of sexual addiction in their lives.
4 Book	Change in life focus.	Ask group members to share how sexual addiction has become a primary motivator, a primary need.
4 Book	Sex addiction cycle and rituals.	No discussion is needed. Just recognize that sex addiction cycles and rituals exist and will be addressed later.
4 Book	Denial.	Ask group members for examples of illogical thinking they use to justify sexual behavior.

From Chapter One of the book:

Page #	**Action:** Read	
4-5 Book	**Primary Topic:** Unwanted Sexual Behaviors Found in the *Diagnostic and Statistical Manual of Mental Disorders, Fourth Edition* (*DSM-IV-TR*).	The purpose of this section is to introduce the behaviors related to sexual addiction that are considered by the mental health profession as disorders.
	Discussion topics:	**Discussion Points:**

| 4-5 Book | Unwanted sexual behaviors. | Ask group members to read this section to themselves. It is enough for group members to understand that paraphilias exist and some members may identify with one or more. However, a discussion of paraphilias at this stage of the program should be done in individual therapy, if needed. |

From Chapter One of the book:

Page #	**Action:** Read and discuss.	
6 Book	**Primary Topic:** Unwanted Sexual Behaviors Not Found in the *DSM-IV-TR*.	The purpose of this section is to introduce the behaviors that are often addressed in sexual addiction therapy but are not considered disorders.
	Discussion topics:	**Discussion Points:**
6 Book	More unwanted sexual behaviors	Ask group members to read this section to themselves. Ask if there are questions. Discuss as needed.

From Chapter One of the book:

Page #	**Action:** Read and discuss.	
6-7 Book	**Primary Topic:** Compulsive Sexual Behaviors.	The purpose of this section is to introduce the compulsive sexual behaviors which are frequently the subject therapy.
	Discussion topics:	**Discussion Points:**
6-7 Book	Masturbation. Pornography. Cybersex. Phone Sex.	Ask group members if they identify with any of the following behaviors. Discussion should be brief but enough to foster awareness.

From Chapter One of the book:

Page #	**Action:** Read and discuss.	
7-13 Book	**Primary Topic:** Underlying Factors of Sexual Addiction.	The purpose of this section is to introduce underlying factors that often lead to or support sexual addiction.

	Discussion topics:	**Discussion Points:**
7 Book	Were you sexually abused as a child or adolescent?	Ask group members how they identify with the following factors. Discussion should be brief but enough to foster awareness.
7 Book	Do you regularly purchase sexually explicit magazines?	
8 Book	Do you regularly pursue online pornography?	
8 Book	Are you often preoccupied with sexual thoughts?	
9 Book	What is the problem? Don't all people have sexual memories?	
9 Book	Does your spouse or significant other ever worry or complain about your sexual behavior?	
9 Book	Can you stop your sexual behavior when you know it's inappropriate?	
10 Book	Do you ever feel badly about your sexual behavior?	
10 Book	Has sexual behavior ever created problems for you or your family?	
10 Book	Do you worry about people finding out about this behavior?	
10 Book	Do you lead a double life?	
11 Book	Do you keep secrets about your sexual or romantic activities from those important to you?	
11 Book	Has your behavior ever emotionally hurt someone?	

11 Book	Are any of your sexual activities against the law (for example, sex with minors or exposure of genitals in public)?	
11 Book	Have you ever felt degraded by your sexual activity?	
11 Book	Do you feel depressed after having sex?	
12 Book	Do you fear sexual intimacy? Do you avoid sex at all costs?	
12 Book	Do you frequently feel remorse, shame, or guilt after a sexual encounter?	
12 Book	Have you ever tried to limit or stop masturbating?	
12 Book	Do you lose your sense of identity or meaning in life without sex or a love relationship?	
13 Book	Does your pursuit of sex or romantic relationships interfere with your spiritual development?	

From Chapter One of the book:

Page #	**Action:** Read and discuss.	
13-14 Book	**Primary Topic:** Insights into Sexual Addiction.	The purpose of this section is to introduce another author's insights into sexual addiction.
	Discussion topics:	**Discussion Points:**
13-14 Book	Insights into sexual addiction.	Ask group members: If they identify with any of the statements? If there are questions? Discuss as needed.

Discuss key points group members learned from this chapter. Insights gained become the fuel for changed behavior.

Handouts: None.

Homework assignment: Read and complete Chapter One of the workbook, *In Search of Recovery: A Christian Man's Guide*

End with a Prayer. (Suggest the Serenity Prayer)

Group Program
Session Four

Goal: Penetrate shame and denial.	Material needed: Workbook, *In Search of Recovery: A Christian Man's Guide*
Objective: Gain deeper understanding of one's addiction.	Chapter: One

Begin with a Prayer

Continue with remaining material from the previous session.

From Chapter One of the workbook:

Page #	Action: Read and discuss.	
3-4 Workbook	Primary Topic: Men's Stories.	The purpose of this section is to introduce other men's stories to help group members understand they did not invent the sexual addiction wheel.
	Discussion topics:	Discussion Points:
3-4 Workbook	Andre's Story. Neil's Story. David's Story. Mike's Story. Ted's Story. Tony's Story. George's Story. James' Story.	Ask group members: If they identify with any of the stories presented? To share their feelings when they identify with another man's story. (Are they relieved to find others have had the same problem?)

From Chapter One of the workbook:

Page #	**Action:** Read, complete the exercises, and discuss.	
4-27 Workbook	**Primary Topic:** How about You?	The purpose of this exercise is for each man to get in touch with the magnitude and impact of his sexual behaviors.
	Discussion topics:	**Discussion Points:**
4-22 Workbook	Pornography. Masturbation. Sexual fantasy and thinking. Sexual encounters. Other sexual activities.	Ask group members: To complete their sexual inventory. To share their answers as they feel comfortable in doing so. If they discovered anything new when they completed their inventory? To share shame or guilt feelings they experienced while completing their inventory. **Note:** Group members generally find completing sex behavioral inventory helpful and revealing. However, for some it is an embarrassing task. As such, it may take time for each man to fully disclose his sexual history. Gaining awareness and facing reality and denial are important tasks for group members. As disclosure progresses, shame will begin to diminish.
23 Workbook	Legality.	Talk about the risks of using a work based computer to view pornography or enter chat rooms.
24-27 Workbook	Your story.	**Note:** This section is for group members whose sexual behavior does not fit one of the listed categories, for example, one of the paraphilias or bestiality.

From Chapter One of the workbook:

Page #	**Action:** Read, complete the exercises, and discuss.	

28-31 Workbook	**Primary Topic:** Sexual Addiction Questions.	The purpose of this section is to explore sexual addiction corollaries as they relate to each man.
	Discussion topics:	**Discussion Points:**
28 Workbook	Have your sexual practices become compulsive and unmanageable?	Ask group members to share past efforts to end acting-out behavior and their results.
28 Workbook	Have you experienced life-damaging consequences as a result of your sexual behavior?	Ask group members: Is isolation a primary consequence? To discuss other consequences including self-loathing, depression, anxiety, anger, despair, pervasive feelings of hopelessness, and broken relationships with family and God.
28 Workbook	Has your sexual addiction caused a change in your life focus?	Ask group members if sexual behavior has become a primary motivator, a primary need.
29 Workbook	Is keeping your sexual behavior a secret very important to you?	Ask group members how secrecy keeps the addicted man bound to addiction.
29 Workbook	Do you fear giving up your best friend, your sexual addiction?	Ask group members if they fear giving up cherished sexual behavior, an old and familiar friend. **Note:** This is an important insight for group members.
29 Workbook	Have you denied that you have a sexual addiction problem?	At this stage several group members are still questioning if they are sexually addicted. Ask group members to share their thinking.
29-31 Workbook	What lies and excuses do you use to continue your sexual behavior?	Ask group members to: Complete the exercises. Share "lies and excuses" they use to justify sexual behavior. **Note:** Post answers to newsprint or a board. It is important for group members to realize that "lies and excuses" facilitate addiction.

From Chapter One of the workbook:

Page #	Action: Read, complete the exercises, and discuss.	
32-34 Workbook	Primary Topic: Am I Sexually Addicted?	The purpose of this section is to penetrate denial.
	Discussion topics:	Discussion Points:
32 Workbook	Am I sexually addicted questions:	Ask group members to: Complete the exercises. Share answers to the question(s) Yes, No, Maybe I am sexually addicted. Why?
33-34 Workbook	I have examined my unwanted sexual behaviors and determined that I want to change . . .	Ask group members to: Complete the exercises. Share their answers. Note: Answers may be unrealistic at this point. The purpose to help group members begin to think about change.

Discuss key points group members learned from this chapter (End of workbook Chapter One). Insights gained become the fuel for changed behavior.

Handouts: None.

Homework Assignment: Read and complete Chapters Two from the book and workbook, *In Search of Recovery: A Christian Man's Guide*

End with a Prayer. (Suggest the Serenity Prayer)

Group Program
Sessions Five and Six

Goal: Penetrating shame by understanding sexual addiction was initially not a choice.	Material needed: book and workbook, *In Search of Recovery: A Christian Man's Guide*
Objective: Gain deeper understanding of one's childhood sexual addiction roots.	Chapter: Two

Begin with a Prayer

Continue with remaining material from the previous session. When completed, begin Chapter Two in the book and workbook, *In Search of Recovery: A Christian Man's Guide*

From Chapter Two of the book and workbook:

Page #	Action: Read, complete the exercises, and discuss.	
15-22 Book	Primary Topic: Sexual Addiction Often Begins in Childhood.	The purpose of this section is to introduce the conditions that often form the root of sexual addiction in a story form.
	Discussion topics:	Discussion Points:
15-18 Book 37-39 Workbook	Jack's Story. Ted's Story. Hank's Story. Art's Story. Simon's Story.	Ask group members to read and consider the conditions that fostered sexual addiction in the men in each vignette. Note: Supplement by reading "Mark's Story" from pages 37-39 of the workbook. The conditions are summarized on page 37 of the workbook.

19-20 Book	Common elements in the above vignettes.	Ask group members to: Identify the conditions that fostered sexual addiction from the vignettes. Discuss the conditions.
37-39 Workbook		**Note:** First use the questions from pages **19-20** in the book and then the exercises from pages **38-39** in the workbook. Use the workbook for discussion purposes.
21-22 Book and **40-43** Workbook	Common elements in your life. Your Story.	Ask group members: To identify the conditions that formed the group members' sexual addiction. To complete the answers to the questions. Allow each group member to present his story. **Note:** First use the questions from pages **21-22** in the book and then the exercises from pages **40-43** in the workbook. Use the workbook for discussion purposes. **Note:** It is common for some group members to have difficulty recalling their story. Hearing other men recall their stories may trigger memories. For some, memories will be unsettling. Memories of experiencing or causing abuse may require individual counseling.

From Chapter Two of the workbook:

Page #	**Action:** Read, complete the exercises, and discuss.	
44 Workbook	**Primary Topic:** Sexual Addiction Can Begin in Teenage or Early Adulthood.	The purpose of this section is to introduce the conditions that form the root of sexual addiction when the addiction begins in teen years or early adulthood.
	Discussion topics:	**Discussion Points:**

44 Workbook	Joshua's Story—an alternative story.	Ask group members to: Identify the conditions that formed Joshua's sexual addiction. Discuss the conditions and how those experienced by Joshua are different from those experienced by children who are exposed to age-inappropriate sexual material or behavior during childhood.
44 Workbook	Your Story—an alternative story.	Ask group members to: Identify the conditions that fostered sexual addiction. Complete the exercises. Discuss the events. **Note:** This section may be passed over if all of the group members experienced childhood exposure.

From Chapter Two of the book:

Page #	**Action:** Read and discuss.	
23-28 Book	**Primary Topic:** Highlight the Origin of Sexual Addiction.	The purposes of this section are to allow more discussion of the origin of sexual addiction and to firmly set in the minds of group members that they did not ask to be sexually addicted. **Note:** Long-term healing is aided by a diminution of shame associated with sexual addiction. Men cannot change what has happened to them, but they can choose, as adults, to stop experiencing pain rooted in childhood.
	Discussion topics:	**Discussion Points:**
23 Book	Age-inappropriate exposure to sexual behavior or material.	Ask group members: What was the consequence of their age-inappropriate exposure? To discuss sexual behavior they adopted subsequently to exposure. How such behavior progressed during teen and adult life. To discuss their feelings when they experienced abuse. **Note:** The age-inappropriate exposure is referred to as a *catalytic event* or a *catalytic story*.

23-25 Book	Family environment and structure.	Ask group members to: Share whether their family environment met their childhood need for affection and emotional nourishment. If not, why not? Assess their family as rigid or chaotic. Share how their family environment contribute to living in isolation? Share if they feel isolated today. Discuss feelings generated by isolation. Discuss how their family environment fed their addiction. Share feelings associated with growing-up in their family. **Note:** Not all men who are exposed to unwanted sexual material or acts go on to have a difficulty with adult sexual addiction. The relationship between the child and parent makes a significant difference.
25-26 Book	Arousal.	Ask group members to: Share how well they remember their catalytic event. Ask why they can't remember what was served on one's birthday that year—another special occasion. Discuss why the catalytic event was encoded in their brain. (It was one of the defining moments of life.) Discuss feelings associated with arousal . . . excitement, shame, guilt, confusion, etc.
26-27 Book	Feelings of shame, guilt, and depression.	Ask group members to: Discuss the difference between feeling guilty and ashamed. Relate why their addiction fostered feelings of shame, guilt, and depressed mood. Why is loving marital sex not accompanied by similar feelings? Discuss how shame fuels sexual compulsivity (need to medicate depressed mood and other negative feelings). Discuss if depressed mood plays a role in their lives.
27 Book	Learned model in childhood repeated in adulthood.	Ask group members if they repeat behaviors first began in childhood? Why?

27-28 Book	Richard's Story.	Ask group members if: They identify with the conditional love experienced by Richard? Sexual behaviors were passed down from one generation to the next in their family? They will pass their sexual addiction on to their children? Ask group members: To share memories of conditional love from their families of origin. To describe how it felt to be loved conditionally. In what way do group members love their children conditionally?

Discuss key points group members learned from this chapter (end of the workbook Chapter Two) Insights gained become the fuel for changed behavior.

Handouts: None.

Homework Assignment: Read and complete Chapters Three from the book and workbook, *In Search of Recovery: A Christian Man's Guide*

End with a Prayer. (Suggest the Serenity Prayer)

Group Program
Sessions Seven, Eight, and Nine

Goal: Understanding the sobriety challenge.	**Material needed:** book and workbook, *In Search of Recovery: A Christian Man's Guide*
Objective: Gain deeper understanding of the complexity of sexual addiction.	**Chapter:** Three

Begin with a Prayer

Continue with remaining material from the previous session. When completed, begin Chapter Three in the book and workbook, *In Search of Recovery A Christian man's Guide*

From Chapter Three of the book and workbook:

Page #	Action: Read and discuss.	
29-31 Book	**Primary Topic:** Brain Indoctrination.	The purpose of this section is to explain how sexual addiction has changed the brain.
	Discussion topics:	**Discussion Points:**
29 Book	Habit.	Ask group members: If they habitually repeat their sexual thinking, fantasy, and behavior? To discuss how sex becomes the addict's number one focus—his number one need.
51-53 Workbook		**Note:** Supplement with the exercises under, "Altering the brain and forming a habit," from pages **51-53** of the workbook.

30 Book	Sexual fantasies.	Ask group members: To discuss how sexual thinking and fantasy precede acting out. If they agree that their sexual fantasies are part of their brain's indoctrination and serve as a launching platform for acting out? Why not just stop sexual thinking and fantasy if it is the precursor to acting out? Discuss why it is difficult to stop.
54-57 Workbook		**Note:** Supplement with exercises under, "Sexual Fantasies," from pages **54-57** of the workbook. Ultimately, a commitment to change involves gaining control over the mind. These materials can be powerful and are a good supplement to the book. Ask group members to: Examine how sexual fantasies play a key role in continuing acting-out behaviors. Share their answers to the questions in the exercise.
30-31 Book	Altering the brain.	Ask group members: If their brain now considers repetitive sexual stimulation normal? Why does the brain encourage repetition of sexual activity to generate pleasurable feelings? To discuss why the brain remembers euphoria related to orgasm. What is the role of endorphins?
31 Book	Association of systems.	Ask group members to share and name the associations that precede their acting out.
57-59 Workbook	Your sexually acting-out environment.	Ask group members: How their environment supports their acting-out behavior. To name their environmental triggers.
57 Workbook	Jude's Story.	Ask group members in what way do they identify with Jude's Story.
58-59 Workbook	Your Story.	Ask group members to complete the exercise and share how their environment supports acting-out behavior.

From Chapter Three of the book:

Page #	**Action:** Read and discuss.	
31-34 Book	**Primary Topic:** Isolation.	The purpose of this section is to explain how isolation is toxic to the sexually addicted man.
	Discussion topics:	**Discussion Points:**
31-32 Book	Hiding behind the mask.	Ask group members: What does it mean to hide behind a mask for the sexually addicted man? What would taking off the mask look like? How does one become vulnerable, that is, come out of isolation by sharing the "real me?"
32 Book	Loneliness to isolation.	Ask group members: Is the price of isolation loneliness? How does childhood isolation spill over into adulthood? If they feel lonely in their marriage? How can feelings of loneliness be changed?
32-33 Book	Codependency.	Ask group members: What does it mean to be in a codependent relationship? Would their marriage relationship be termed codependent? If so, why? **Note:** Discuss the text fully. Addressing codependent behavior is important to long-term healing.
33 Book	Sex to medicate pain.	Ask group members: If they use sex to deal with life's problems and pain? What life conditions are medicated? Is medicating pain through sex linked to isolation?
34 Book	Sexual abuse as a child.	Ask group members: To briefly discuss any new insights into how the combination of age-inappropriate sexual stimulus and dysfunctional family life is a formula for isolation and addiction. If it is time to give up the childhood mode and make an adult decision to change? What would it look like to come out of isolation?

From Chapter Three of the workbook:

Page #	Action: Read, do exercises and discuss.	
59-63 Workbook	**Primary Topic:** Acting-out Ritual.	The purpose of this section is to explain how sexual addiction is based on predictable ritual patterns.
	Discussion topics:	**Discussion Points:**
59-60 Workbook	Tom's acting-out ritual.	Ask group members to: Read Tom's acting-out ritual. Identify points where Tom could have ended his ritual.
60-63 Workbook	Your acting-out rituals.	Ask group members to: Complete the exercises (most men have multiple rituals). Share their acting-out rituals. Examine early points in the ritual(s) where an intervention could be successful. Express their feelings at each step of their ritual.
36-38 Book		**Note:** Supplement by reading, "Greg's Story," from pages **36-38** of the book. Establish an understanding that most sexual behavior is accompanied by ritual. Ultimately the goal is to recognize the early steps of the ritual and to reject them.

From Chapter Three of the workbook:

Page #	Action: Read, complete the exercises and discuss.	
64-68 Workbook	**Primary Topic:** Sex Addiction Cycle.	The purpose of this section is to explain the sexual addict's acting-out cycle.
	Discussion topics:	**Discussion Points:**
64 Workbook	Sex Addiction Cycle	Ask group members to read the introduction to Sex Addiction Cycle.

65 Workbook	Initial phase—life condition.	Ask group members to: Read the initial phase—life condition. Record and discuss one's life conditions and identify the reason why this is the beginning of the acting-out cycle. What changes in feelings or mood do they identify at the beginning of phase one? Identify early feelings or changes in mood that could be addressed to preclude the acting-out cycle.
66 Workbook	Phase two—reaction to life condition.	Ask group members to: Read phase two—reaction to life condition. Record and discuss one's reaction to one's life condition. Identify the reason this reaction contributes to the repetition of the acting-out cycle.
67 Workbook	Phase three—acting-out.	Ask group members to: Read phase three—acting out. Disclose an example of their acting-out rituals.
68 Workbook	Phase four—reconciliation	Ask group members to: Read phase four—reconciliation. Record and discuss one's feelings of shame and guilt. Record thinking that allows one to reject feelings of shame and guilt in order to repeat the cycle. **Note:** Establish an understanding that sexually addicted men repeat their acting-out cycles. Ultimately the goal is to recognize early steps within the cycle and choose alternative thinking and environments to reject repeating the acting-out cycle. Men seeking recovery often put more time between their addiction cycles. Unfortunately, increasing time between acting-out behaviors only constitutes longer cycles, not recovery.

Discuss key points group members learned from this chapter (end of the workbook Chapter Three). Insights gained become the fuel for changed behavior.

Handouts: None.

Homework Assignment: Read and complete Chapters Four from the book and workbook, *In Search of Recovery: A Christian Man's Guide*

End with a Prayer. (Suggest the Serenity Prayer)

Group Program
Sessions Ten, Eleven, and Twelve

Goal: Seeing the whole sexual addiction picture.	**Material needed:** book and workbook, *In Search of Recovery: A Christian Man's Guide*
Objective: Gain a deeper understanding of the host of conditions that contribute to or support sexual addiction.	**Chapter:** Four

Begin with a Prayer

Continue with remaining material from the previous session. When completed, begin Chapter Four in the book and workbook, *In Search of Recovery: A Christian Man's Guide*

From Chapter Four of the book and workbook:

Page #	**Action:** Read and discuss.	
39-42 Book **71-79** Workbook	**Primary Topic:** Role of Anger.	The purpose of this section is to understand that anger is a companion of the sexually addicted man. Anger is a product of acting out, and, conversely, anger contributes to acting out. Often anger has, as does sexual addiction, it roots in childhood child/parent relationships.
	Discussion topics:	**Discussion Points:**
71-72 Workbook	Childhood emotional nourishment.	Ask group members if they identify with any of the characterizations of fathers?
72 Workbook	Ely's Story.	Ask group members to comment on the type of love Ely's father had for Ely.

72-74 Workbook	Your family of origin.	Ask group members to: Complete the exercises and think about what it was like growing-up in their families. Share and discuss answers and insights to the questions. Share feelings related to their relationship with their fathers. Share the impact and feelings of not feeling valued.
74-77 Workbook	Childhood messages.	Ask group members to: Complete the exercises and think about the messages received from family members during childhood. Share and discuss answers to the questions. Share the feelings these messages generated. How did the messages govern the assessment of one's self worth? Share how deflating messages foster isolation and addiction. What messages do group members send to their children?
39-40 Book **71** Workbook **78-79** Workbook	Role of Anger. Childhood abuse.	Explore the connection between anger and childhood family experience and/or abuse. **Note:** Supplement by reading, "Sexual Iceberg," from page **71** of the workbook. **Note:** Supplement by completing the exercises under, "Role of Anger," from page **78-79** of the workbook.
40 Book	Ralph's Story.	Ask group members: What is the lesson presented in Ralph's Story? If their anger is proportional to the importance of events? What would it mean to realize one is not a bad person but a person who is struggling with a bad problem?

41-42 Book	Rules in the head. Sean's Story.	Ask group members: If they have rules in their heads related to performance of others (wife, children, parents, work associates, etc.)? Give examples and discuss. If others know they are being held accountable? What is the outcome of not being in control of one's environment?
42 Book	Anger at God.	Ask group members: If they ever perceived themselves as being angry at God? To characterize their anger at God—is it helpful or defeating? Describe a reasonable expectation of God in one's life journey.
42 Book	Anger alters mood.	Ask group members: If they have experienced mood alteration during anger or rage? How could anger substitute for acting-out sexually?

From Chapter Four of the book and workbook:

Page #	**Action:** Read and discuss.	
43-45 Book	**Primary Topic:** Role of Anxiety.	The purpose of this section is to understand that anxiety is often a companion of the sexually addicted man. Anxiety is both a product of and a contributor to acting-out behavior.
	Discussion topics:	**Discussion Points:**
43 Book	Sexual anxiety	Ask group members: Does anxiety create sexual tension in their bodies? What impact does anxiety have in fostering addiction?
80-82 Workbook		**Note:** Supplement by completing the exercises under, "The Role of Anxiety," from pages **80-82** of the workbook.
43 Book	Barry's Story.	Ask group members if they have difficulty facing normal activities until they masturbate to relieve anxiety.

43-44 Book	Situational anxiety.	Ask group members to describe situations that cause anxiety in their lives. Is acting out a solution to situational anxiety?
43-44 Book	Todd's Story.	Ask group members if they identify with Todd? How could Todd deal with his situational anxiety?
44-45 Book	Chronic anxiety.	Ask group members if living with anxiety has become a way of life?
44-45 Book	Mack's Story.	Ask group members if they identify with Mack?
45 Book	Treatment.	Ask group members to discuss the pros and cons of taking medication to control anxiety.

From Chapter Four of the book and workbook:

Page #	**Action:** Read and discuss.	
45-51 Book	**Primary Topic:** Role of Depressed Mood.	The purpose of this section is to understand that depressed mood is often a companion of the sexually addicted man. Depressed mood is both a product of and a contributor to acting-out behavior.
	Discussion topics:	**Discussion Points:**
45-49 Book	Chronic depressed mood.	Read and discuss the "Role of depressed Mood," from pages **45-49** in the book. Ask group members: If they experience long periods of low-grade depressed mood? What impact does depressed mood have in fostering addiction?
82-84 Workbook		**Note:** Supplement by reading and completing the exercises under, "The Role of Depressed Mood," from pages **82-84** of the workbook
46-48 Book	Addict's Life Scale	Ask group members: To discuss the concepts. If they identify with the life scale values?

85-86 Workbook	Your Life Scale	Ask group members: To complete their life scales. To discuss how the life scale relates to their lives. To talk about their feelings associated with each level of their life scale How would they characterize their depressed mood. At what scale value do they live? If their depressed mood is destructive? To discuss the consequences of living with depressed mood in their lives. To discuss the pros and cons of taking medication to stabilize mood.
50 Book	Next steps.	Ask group members to discuss the steps they can take to come out of their depressed mood.
50-51 Book	Pete's Story.	Ask group members: How they could change their lives to live at 40? Record on large sheets of paper or on a board. To share insights gained from Pete's Story.

From Chapter Four of the workbook:

Page #	**Action:** Read, complete exercises, and discuss.	
86-88 Workbook	**Primary Topic:** Role of Isolation.	The purpose of this section is to understand that isolation and loneliness are breeding grounds for depressed mood and sexual addiction.
	Discussion topic:	**Discussion Points:**
86-88 Workbook	Isolation and loneliness.	Ask group members to: Complete the exercises and think about what it is like to frequently experience isolation and loneliness. Share answers and insights to the questions. Share feelings related to isolation and loneliness. Share the impact of isolation and loneliness in fostering addiction. Share how men can come out of isolation. Record on large paper or a board.

From Chapter Four of the workbook:

Page #	**Action:** Read and discuss.	
90 Workbook	**Primary Topic:** Keep in Mind.	The purpose of this section is to review the tenants of this chapter.
	Discussion topic.	**Discussion Points:**
90 Workbook	Share insights.	Ask group members to read and share insights.

Discuss key points group members learned from this chapter (end of the workbook Chapter Four). Insights gained become the fuel for changed behavior.

Handouts: None.

Homework Assignment: Read and complete Chapter Five from the book and workbook, *In Search of Recovery: A Christian Man's Guide*

End with a Prayer. (Suggest the Serenity Prayer)

Group Program
Sessions Thirteen and Fourteen

Goal: Reveal hope.	**Material needed:** book and workbook, *In Search of Recovery A Christian: Man's Guide*
Objective: Gain deeper understanding of how the Lord loved other noted sinners. If He loved them, He can love the sexually addicted man.	**Chapter:** Five

Begin with a Prayer

Continue with remaining material from the previous session. When completed, begin Chapter Five in the book and workbook, *In Search of Recovery: A Christian Man's Guide*

From Chapter Four of the book and workbook:

Page #	Action: Read, complete the exercises, and discuss.	
91-96 Workbook	**Primary Topic:** Is There Hope?	The purpose of this section is to understand that hope is available for the sexually addicted man. God does not give up on us.
	Discussion topics:	**Discussion Points:**
91 Workbook	Salvation history.	Ask group members to read and complete the exercises for each historical person presented as part of salvation history. Ask group members: Are we bad men, or are we just dealing with a bad problem? What is a bad person? Why would it be harmful to accept the conclusion, "I am a bad person?"

91-93 Workbook	King David.	Ask group members to ponder this: King David was a sinful man, but the Lord chose him to be at the head of Jesus' lineage. What does that imply for us?
93 Workbook	Apostle Peter.	Ask group members to ponder this: Peter was a sinful man, but the Lord chose him to be the rock upon which He built His church. What does that imply for us?
93-96 Workbook	Apostle Paul.	Ask group members: To ponder this: Paul was a sinful man, but the Lord chose him to take the Word to the gentiles. What does that imply for us? Discuss the nature of the thorn in Paul's side. Could Paul's thorn have been addiction? If so, what does that imply for us?
96 Workbook **56-57** Book	Change the dance.	Ask group members if David, Peter, and Paul could change, can addicted men do the same? Is God's grace sufficient for us? **Note:** Supplement by reading and discussing, "Sonny's Story and "Treatment goals," from pages **56-57** of the book.

Discuss key points group members learned from this chapter (end of the workbook Chapter Five) Insights gained become the fuel for changed behavior.

Handouts: None.

Homework Assignment: Read and complete Chapters Six from the book and workbook, *In Search of Recovery: A Christian Man's Guide*

End with a Prayer. (Suggest the Serenity Prayer)

Group Program
Sessions Fifteen and Sixteen

Goal: Awareness of choice.	**Material needed:** book and workbook, *In Search of Recovery: A Christian Man's Guide*
Objective: Gain deeper awareness of the possibility of changing the sexual addiction dance.	**Chapter:** Six

Begin with a Prayer

Continue with remaining material from the previous session. When completed, begin Chapter Six in the book and workbook, *In Search of Recovery: A Christian Man's Guide*

From Chapter Six of the book and workbook:

Page #	**Action:** Read and discuss.	
62 Book	**Primary Topic:** Awareness Leads to Choice.	The purpose of this section is to understand that what has been learned to date serves as a platform to change the sexual addiction dance.
	Discussion topic:	**Discussion Points**

61-62 Book	Awareness leads to choices.	Ask group members to: Discuss why awareness leads to choice. Do members of the group agree or disagree? Ponder this question: While I did not ask to become sexually addicted, is it time to make an adult decision to change my sexual addiction dance?
99-107 Workbook	Summary Review. Affect on my life. The origin of my addiction. Factors that keep me addicted. Role of anger. Role of anxiety. Role of low-grade depression. Role of isolation. Exceptions.	Ask group members to: Complete the exercises and think about the totality of what keeps each man addicted. Share and discuss any new insight gained or additional information discovered since recording one sexual inventory in Chapter One. Share feelings after completing each exercise. Share insights gained from reviewing the full sexual addiction picture. Answer the question, "Am I ready to move on?"

From Chapter Six of the book and workbook:

Page #	**Action:** Read, complete the exercises, and discuss.	
62-66 Book	**Primary Topic:** Changing the Dance—New Steps.	The purpose of this section is to begin identifying the essential new steps needed to change the sexual addiction dance.
	Discussion topics:	**Discussion Points:**

62-66 Book	Changing the Dance—New Steps. Commitment. Awareness as part of commitment. Bill's Story.	Ask group members to: Read and think about what changing the sexual addiction dance means. Discuss the difference between "white-knuckling" and a "high-level commitment." Describe "white-knuckling" efforts that are not working. Describe what a "high-level commitment" would look like. Discuss what an "irrevocable decision" means to the sexually addicted man. Discuss the handout, *Stash*. Discuss the meaning of "stash." Share if they are willing to take a recovery step by trashing all stash. Share insights gained from this section.
107-109 Workbook		**Note:** Supplement by completing the exercises, "Changing the Dance" from pages **107-109** of the workbook.
66 Book	Recognize that addiction causes more pain than pleasure.	Ask group members to: Read and compare long-term pain of guilt and shame to the short-term pleasure of acting out. Discuss the difference between long-term pain and a short-term pleasure. Answer the question: Is my equation out of balance? Answer the question: If my pain is greater than my pleasure, why would I want to continue to accept that pain? Share insights gained from this section.
109-110 Workbook		**Note:** Supplement by completing the exercise, "Recognize that addiction causes more pain than pleasure," from pages **109-110** of the workbook.

66-67 Book	Address Environmental Temptation. Jim's Story. Jay's Story. Matt's Story.	Ask group members to: Read and think about how environmental temptations keep men trapped in sexual addiction. Discuss what environmental factors need to be addressed when a high-level commitment is made to end sexually addictive thinking, fantasy, and behavior. Discuss each story as it relates to addressing environmental temptation. Read and think about how environmental temptations keep group members trapped in sexual addiction.
110 Workbook		**Note:** Supplement by completing the exercises, "Address Environmental Temptation" from page **110** of the workbook.

Discuss key points group members learned from this chapter (end of the workbook Chapter Six). Insights gained become the fuel for changed behavior.

Handouts: Stash.

Homework Assignment: Read and complete Chapters Seven from the book and workbook, *In Search of Recovery: A Christian Man's Guide.*

End with a Prayer. (Suggest the Serenity Prayer)

Group Program
Sessions Seventeen and Eighteen

Goal: Choosing a healthy lifestyle.	**Material needed:** book and workbook, *In Search of Recovery: A Christian Man's Guide*
Objective: Understand choices that constitute a healthy lifestyle free of sex addiction.	**Chapter:** Seven

Begin with a Prayer

Continue with remaining material from the previous session. When completed, begin Chapter Seven in the book and workbook, *In Search of Recovery: A Christian Man's Guide*

From Chapter Seven of the book:

Page #	Action: Read and discuss.	
69-80 Book	**Topic:** What is a Healthy Life Style?	The purpose of this section is to define four elements of a healthy lifestyle.
	Discussion topic:	**Discussion Points:**

69-80 Book	Why is changing one's life style important?	Ask group members to project how a healthier lifestyle would: Impact sexually addictive behavior. Raise depressed mood Enable a new relationship with God. Enable feelings of peace and joy. Reduce feelings of shame. Ask group members: Why is a healthy lifestyle essential to sexual addiction recovery? What would a healthy lifestyle look like? How would a healthy lifestyle complement a high-level commitment to end sexual thinking, fantasy, and behavior? What are the benefits of living a healthy life style?

From Chapter Seven of the book and workbook:

Page #	**Action:** Read and discuss.	
69-73 Book	**Primary Topic:** Coming Out of Isolation.	The purpose of this section is to explore the steps that define coming out of isolation.
70 Book **113-115** Workbook	Coming out of isolation by cultivating a strong male friendship.	Ask group members: Why does coming out of isolation include cultivating a strong male friendship? To discuss whether cultivating a strong male friendship is easy or difficult. Why? Share insights gained from this section. **Note:** Supplement by completing the exercises under, "Coming Out of Isolation," and "Coming out of isolation by cultivating a strong male friendship," from pages **113-115** of the workbook.
70-71 Book **115-116** Workbook	Coming out of isolation by improving family relationships.	Ask group members why coming out of isolation includes improving family relationships. **Note:** Supplement by completing the exercises under, "Coming out of isolation by improving family relationships," from pages **115-116** of the workbook.

71-73 Book 116-118 Workbook	Coming out of isolation by improving relationships with spouse and children.	Ask group members why coming out of isolation includes improving relationships with one's spouse and children. **Note:** Supplement by completing the exercises under, "Coming out of isolation by improving relationships with spouse and children," from pages **116-118** of the workbook.
71-72 Book	I know that I have intimacy in my marriage when . . .	Ask group members: Why is fostering non-sexual intimacy essential to improving family relationships? What is the difference in relationship building between non-sexual intimacy and sexual intimacy?

From Chapter Seven of the book and workbook:

Page #	**Action:** Read and discuss.	
73-74 Book	**Primary Topic:** Giving-up Depressed Mood	The purpose of this section is to explore how giving-up depressed mood supports sexual addiction recovery.
	Discussion topic:	**Discussion Points:**
73-74 Book 118-121 Workbook	Choose to take steps to live at 40.	Ask group members: Why is giving up a depressed mood essential to sexual addiction recovery? What would living life closer to 40 look like? Answer the question: What activities would I incorporate into my life to live closer to 40? How would giving up a depressed mood complement a high-level commitment to end sexual thinking, fantasy, and behavior? What are the consequences of giving up a depressed mood? **Note:** Supplement by completing the exercises under, "Giving-up depressed mood," and Choose to take steps to live at 40," from pages **118-121** of the workbook.

From Chapter Seven of the book and workbook:

Page #	Action: Read and discuss.	
74 Book	**Primary Topic:** Put God First.	The purpose of this section is to explore why a changed relationship with God is an essential sexual addiction recovery step.
	Discussion topic:	**Discussion Points:**
74 Book	Asking God to come into one's life.	Ask group members: Why is a changed relationship with God an essential step in overcoming sexual addiction recovery? What would a changed relationship with God look like? How would a changed relationship with God complement a high-level commitment to end sexual thinking, fantasy, and behavior? What are the consequences of a changed relationship with God?
121-123 Workbook		**Note:** Supplement by completing the exercises under, "A Close Relationship with God," and "Change Your Relationship with God," from pages **121-123** of the workbook

From Chapter Seven of the book and workbook:

Page #	Action: Read and discuss.	
74-75 Book	**Primary Topic:** Develop a Support Network	The purpose of this section is to explore how an effective support program is an essential recovery step in overcoming sexual addiction.
	Discussion topic:	**Discussion Points:**

74-75 Book	Twelve-step program and accountability.	Ask group members: Why is it essential to develop a network to support sexual addiction recovery? How would a support network complement a high-level commitment to end sexual thinking, fantasy, and behavior? What would a support network look like? What insights were gained from this section? If they attend one or more sex addiction Twelve Step Programs? How frequent do they attend Twelve Step programs? Do they have an accountability partner? Describe the relationship.
123-124 Workbook		**Note:** Supplement by completing the exercises under, "Develop a Support Network" from pages **123-124** of the workbook

From Chapter Seven of the book:

Page #	**Action:** Read and discuss.	
75-78 Book	**Primary Topic:** Interventions.	The purpose of this section is to provide interventions that men have found useful in times of temptation.
	Discussion topics:	**Discussion Points:**
75-78 Book	Interventions and planning ahead.	Ask group members to: Choose interventions that would support their recovery and explain why. Discuss how the application of interventions differs before and after a high-level commitment. Prepare two cards and share the contents of these cards.

From Chapter Seven of the book:

Page #	**Action:** Read and discuss.	
79-80 Book	**Primary Topic:** New Behaviors in Place of Old Behaviors.	The purpose of this section is to suggest that, on the road to recovery, it is easier and more effective to adopt new behaviors, rather than "white-knuckle" the removal of old behaviors.

	Discussion topics:	Discussion Points:
79-80 Book	New Behaviors in Place of Old Behaviors.	Ask group members: Why is it more prudent to introduce new behaviors in one's life, rather concentrating on backing off old behaviors? What new behaviors support sexual addiction recovery for each man? What insights were gained from this section?
79 Book	Jude's Story. George's Story.	What new behaviors did Jude and George introduce to change their sexual addiction dance?
79 Book	Backing off behaviors.	Ask group members: What behaviors would they find easier to give up? What behaviors would they find difficult to give up?
79-80 Book	Glen's Story.	Ask group members what behaviors Glen found easier to give up. How does this help the sexually addicted man?

Discuss key points group members learned from this chapter (end of the workbook, Chapter Seven). Insights gained become the fuel for changed behavior.

Handouts: None.

Homework Assignment: Read and complete Chapters Eight from the book and workbook, *In Search of Recovery: A Christian Man's Guide*

End with a Prayer. (Suggest the Serenity Prayer)

Group Program
Session Nineteen

Goal: Choose God as a companion on the recovery journey.	**Material needed:** book and workbook, *In Search of Recovery: A Christian Man's Guide*
Objective: Understand the road to recovery goes through a deeper relationship with God.	**Chapter:** Eight

Begin with a Prayer

Continue with remaining material from the previous session. When completed, begin Chapter Eight in the book and workbook, *In Search of Recovery: A Christian Man's Guide*

From Chapter Eight of the book:

Page #	**Action:** Read and discuss.	
81-88 Book	**Primary Topic:** Relationship with God.	The purpose of this section is to explore why recovery is deepened through a relationship with God.
	Discussion topics:	**Discussion Points:**

81-82 Book	Relationship with God and Dave's Story.	Ask group members: Why is a healthy relationship with God essential to sexual addiction recovery? What would a healthy relationship with God look like? How would a healthy relationship with God foster a high-level commitment to end sexual thinking, fantasy, and behavior? What are the consequences of a close relationship with God? What insights were gained from Dave's Story? Ask group members to: Consider how each man can change addiction into grace. Describe the hole in their soul.
82-83 Book	What does my addiction have to do with God?	Ask group members: What would it mean to come to depend on God as one's greatest need, rather than depending on sex? How would a blessed relationship with God help the addict to come out of isolation?
83-84 Book	Jason's Story.	Ask group members: To discuss the transition Jason made in his life, both in changing his addiction dance and in his relationship with God. Why did nothing work for Jason until he made the decision to turn to God? What insights were gained from Jason's Story?
84-85 Book	Andy's Story.	Ask group members: Why did hitting bottom and turning to God happen at the same time for Andy? What insights were gained from Andy's Story?
85-86 Book	Bob's Story.	Ask group members: To discuss the messages Bob shared with Andy. To discuss why Bob had to realize that he was a good person, despite being in prison. Why are we not "trash" to God, despite being sexually addicted? How can God use us? What insights were gained from Bob's Story?

86-87 Book	Committed and genuine relationship with God.	Ask group members: What is a committed and genuine relationship with God? How is a committed and genuine relationship with God different than just going to church each Sunday? Why is a committed and genuine relationship with God like finding the Holy Grail?

From Chapter Eight of the book:

Page #	**Action:** Read and discuss.	
87 Book	**Primary Topic:** Addiction and Grace.	The purpose of this section is to understand that grace is the only hope for dealing with sexual addiction.
	Discussion topic:	**Discussion Points:**
87 Book	Turning addiction and grace.	Ask group members: Why is grace the only hope for dealing with sexual addiction? How can each man turn addiction into grace? What insights were gained from this section?

From Chapter Eight of the book:

Page #	**Action:** Read and discuss.	
87-88 Book	**Primary Topic:** Surrender.	The purpose of this section is to understand that surrendering to the will of God gives power to the sexually addicted man.
	Discussion topic:	**Discussion Points:**
87-88 Book	Surrender one's will to God.	Ask group members: Why does surrendering to the will of God give power to the sexually addicted man? How does surrendering freedom result in becoming truly free? What insights were gained from this section?

Discuss key points group members learned from this chapter.

Handouts: Distribute the exercise, *Prepared to Live a Changed Life* exercise, Appendix B to group members.

Homework Assignment: Read and complete, *Prepared to Live a Changed Life* exercise. Ask the group to be prepared to discuss their answers in the next session.

End with a Prayer. (Suggest the Serenity Prayer)

Group Program
Session Twenty

Goal: Commitment to change.	Material needed: *Preparing to Live a Changed Life* document, Appendix B.
Objective: Understand what a continuing commitment to end sexual addiction looks like.	Chapter: The rest of your life.

Begin with a Prayer

Continue with remaining material from the previous session. When completed, begin working with the *Preparing to Live a Changed Life* exercise.

Preparing to Live a Changed Life.

Ask group members to:

- Share answers from the "change" part of the exercise.

- Discuss why they chose their answers.

- Select three leading changes they plan to address. Limit the focus at this time. If group members can remain committed to three changes, progress will be significant. Some important change items are: come out of isolation, live a healthy lifestyle, maintain a high-level commitment, and deepen one's relationship with God. Group members may wish to address one or more of these in different ways.

- Discuss insights gained from this exercise.

Ask group members to:

- Address the question: "If I am healed, what will I have to give up?"

- Share answers and why each chose their answers.

- Discuss fears of giving up sexual thinking, fantasies, and behaviors that they have lived with for so many years.

- Share how they will keep themselves accountable to live a changed life.

Discuss next steps:

This program is only the beginning of the healing journey. For most men, the journey will take several years and perhaps even the rest of one's life. It is essential for each group member to have a continuing support program.

Ask group members to discuss:

- Attending Sex Addicts Anonymous or another Twelve Step program (See Appendix A: Counseling and Support Programs in the book).

- Reading (See Appendix A: Counseling and Support Programs in the book).

- Maintaining an accountability partner.

- Continuing individual or group therapy.

- Initiating marital therapy.

- Enabling spirituality in one's life.

- Attending specialized treatment programs.

Handouts: None.

Homework Assignment: Continue to attend Twelve Step programs, meet frequently with one's accountability partner, and continue a counseling relationship for times in need.

End with a Prayer. (Suggest the Serenity Prayer)

AMEN: May you and your group members be blessed.

Appendix A: Trash Stash

There are many changes you may chose to make as you journey toward recovery, and they will come in due time. There is, however, a significant step you can take today that will both serve to make a statement of commitment as well as be a positive step that can reduce your acting-out behavior.

The first step is to "trash stash." Sexually addicted men frequently pledge to stop their acting-out behavior. However, most do not get rid of the crutches that facilitate acting out. Stash is the hidden pornographic magazine, the computer URLs that lead to pornography, or the telephone number which the addicted man keeps in case of temptation or sexual urge to act out.

Trashing stash is a firm commitment to remove all lust traps in one's possession. It doesn't mean getting rid of some or most on one's stash, it means getting rid of *all* of it. A commitment to remove stash is not easily made. It means parting with the "keys to the addiction car." Parting with stash is not recovery but an early step toward recovery.

Examples of stash include: computer and access to the Internet; phone sex numbers; pornographic videos, magazines, and CD's; articles of clothing; and sex toys. Your commitment to trash your stash includes a plan to remove or destroy stash.

Complete the exercise:

My Stash is:

1.

_____

_____

2.

_____

_____

3.

_____

_____

My commitment plan is:

1.

_____

_____

2.

_____

_____

3.

_____

_____

Appendix B: Preparing to Live a Changed Life

Choosing a journey free of sex addiction involves changes in how you think, feel, and behave. Although healing ultimately brings a better life, it also threatens to permanently alter life as you have known it. Your relationships, your position in the world, even your sense of identity may change. Old coping patterns may no longer work. When you make the commitment to heal, you risk losing much of what is familiar. As a result, one part of you may want to heal while another resists change.

To prepare to accept change, it is a good idea to cognitively acknowledge where change is likely to take place. Take a few minutes to think about parts of your life that may change as you heal. Then fill out the following change inventory. Start with the areas that are most important to you.

If I live my commitment to heal, the following will probably change:

How my feelings may change (entitlement, shame, guilt, anger, anxiety, depressed mood, attitudes, beliefs, self-image):

1. _____

2. _____

3. _____

4. _____

5. _____

6. _____

How I will change behaviors related to isolation (addiction cycle/addiction ritual/fantasies):

1. _____

2. _____

3. _____

4. _____

How my lifestyle will change (habits, patterns, leisure-time activities, types of friends, efforts to live more often at "40"):

1. _____

2. _____

3. _____

4. _____

5. _____

6. _____

How my relationship with my partner or significant relationship will change:

1. _____

2. _____

3. _____

4. _____

How my relationships will change with my children, siblings, parents, friends:

1. _____

2. _____

3. _____

4. _____

How my continuing recovery program will change (Twelve Step program, counseling, accountability partner, strong male friend):

1. _____

2. _____

3. _____

4. _____

How my spirituality will change:

1. _____

2 _____

3. _____

4. _____

How areas of my life might change:

1. _____

2. _____

3. _____

4. _____

Look over the lists you have made. Put a check mark next to three items where change is likely to occur first. Your commitment should start with these items. As you grow, return to your inventory and add other items that you wish to address in your life.

Also, identify some of your potential losses. Without too much thinking, fill in the following sentences—as many times as you can: (Example: If I healed, I'd have to give up:
    People feeling sorry for me
    Blaming my parents for my problems
    Feeling that I am not worthy of God's love, etc.

Of the things you would have to give up—include such items as fantasies, "stash" (hidden porn magazines, reserved URL's), isolation behaviors, etc.

If healed, I'd have to give up

_____

_____

If healed, I'd have to give up

_____

_____

If healed, I'd have to give up

_____

_____

If healed, I'd have to give up

_____

_____

If healed, I'd have to give up

_____

_____

If healed, I'd have to give up

_____

_____